One Vegan Mama

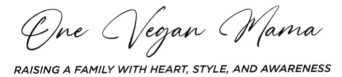

RAISING A FAMILY WITH HEART, STYLE, AND AWARENESS

DEANNA DYLAN

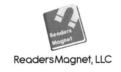

ReadersMagnet, LLC

One Vegan Mama: Raising a Family with Heart, Style, and Awareness
Copyright © 2023 by *Deanna Dylan*

Published in the United States of America
ISBN   Paperback: 979-8-89091-021-9
ISBN   Hardback: 979-8-89091-022-6
ISBN   eBook: 979-8-89091-023-3

All rights reserved. No part of this publication may be reproduced, stored in a retrieval system or transmitted in any way by any means, electronic, mechanical, photocopy, recording or otherwise without the prior permission of the author except as provided by USA copyright law.

The opinions expressed by the author are not necessarily those of ReadersMagnet, LLC.

ReadersMagnet, LLC
10620 Treena Street, Suite 230 | San Diego, California, 92131 USA
1.619. 354. 2643 | www.readersmagnet.com

Book design copyright © 2023 by ReadersMagnet, LLC. All rights reserved.

Cover design by Tifanny Curaza
Interior design by Dorothy Lee

TABLE OF CONTENTS

Introduction 7

My Iowa Roots..8

My Road to Veganism 13

Nonvegan Family and Friends 21

How One Affects the Other 25

My Vegan Pregnancy...32

My Vegan Toddler...39

The Traveling Vegan 42

Future Fashion 46

The Perfect Vegan...50

Corporations Can Evolve 53

Vegans and Activism 57

Five Days of Vegan Meals...60

    Bruschetta 67

    Collard Green Wraps...68

    Dea's Cioppino 69

    Gazpacho..71

    Party Noodles 73

    Perfect Puttanesca...75

    Raw Tunot Salad...77

    Stuffed Peppers 78

Tofu Breakfast Scramble 80
Trees and Nuts Salad 82
Vegan Spaghetti Bolognese 83
Ladies Lunching Sandwiches 85
A Few Fun Tricks 86

The Holidays 88
Films 92
Books 93

Introduction

I am one mother who happens to be raising her family vegan. Being vegan isn't a diet; it's a way of looking at the world. It's one of the best decisions I have made in life. It encompasses so many things I want to teach my daughter. I want her to care about her health and well-being. I also want her to care for others and have compassion. I want her to be a critical thinker, not just go with the flow and be a slave to advertising. I want her to be curious about where things come from and to educate herself always. I want her to stand up for what is right and just even if it isn't popular. Being vegan has the potential to teach her all these things and much more.

You don't have to be vegan or even want to be vegan to gain something positive from this book. I am a busy mom, on the go with a husband, daughter, and three dogs depending on me. I know many can relate. I want the best for my family and for them to be good people, doing all they can to infuse beauty into the world. We can all make a difference in our own lives and the lives of others with our everyday choices. We can live wonderful lives without harming others.

Living vegan is not difficult; it's about choices. You don't have to be a saint or a vegan chef or a nutritionist to do it well. It's a step-by-step building blocks sort of thing. If I can do it, anyone can, and I hope my stories and tips will inspire and help you.

My Iowa Roots

Born and Raised on Meat and Potatoes

I was born and raised in the Midwest—the heartland, specifically Des Moines, Iowa—and from a very young age, I loved animals with a passion. I had so many different pets such as cats, dogs, bunnies, fish, hamsters, hermit crabs, and a turtle named Herman. My sisters and I found strays and brought them home often, so we usually had other animals in addition to our pets.

I have many fond memories of my childhood, and I knew I was loved. However, there was another side to my young life. My childhood was very tumultuous, with lots of abusive and damaged people in and out of our lives after my parents divorced. I played tough, but I often felt vulnerable and worried about my life. My animals gave me incredible comfort and unconditional love. I learned early on how much richer life was with love and respect for animals.

I'll never forget the time my family was driving home and my sister Jennifer spotted a cat attacking a small bunny. She screamed, so my mom pulled the car to the side of the road. We ran over and scared the cat away. We ended up with the bunny on a blanket in our garage. There was so much blood, and the bunny was shaking. I don't remember why we didn't take him to the vet, but I sat in the garage with the bunny all night until he died.

I was devastated. I thought if I loved him enough, he could get better. I was a kid and it was a sad life lesson. Still, I knew that for that little bunny, me being there meant something, and that made me feel good.

One eve in my teen years, I was with a friend on our way home in a rainstorm and we found a tiny kitten on the road. I don't know how we even noticed him. Even back then, I must've had radar for animals in need. I took the little one home, and he gave my entire family ringworm and then somehow escaped, and we never saw him again. My mom was not amused by this scenario.

I cared about my pets being happy. I would take my hermit crabs out and try to train them. It was a terrible failure and a nightmare, I am sure, for the little crabs just trying to hide in their shells. I thought they needed my attention.

I used to fill the bathtub to the top so my turtle Herman could have space to swim. My mom would come home and knock on the locked bathroom door. "Deanna, you don't have that damn turtle in the bathtub again, do you?" I got into trouble, but I still did it every chance I got because he loved it. Herman was one of my favorite childhood friends. When he died, I was upset for quite a while. I buried him in the backyard in a purple and white oatmeal box, with a map, so if we ever moved, I could dig him up and take him with us.

I loved all my animals, even Blackie, the cat that had numerous litters of kittens in my toy box. It was the '70s and my sisters and I all had long hair down to our waists, bell-bottomed jeans on, and lots of freedom to roam.

Our animals had the same liberty, especially the cats. I don't remember hearing anything about spay and neuter or keeping them in the house. Everything was wild and free. It was such a different time.

I was this kid with a huge heart for animals, yet Chicken McNuggets were one of my favorite foods. We frequented McDonald's drive-through, and getting pizza with extra cheese delivered from Pizza Hut was a special treat. I also loved salami and lots of other meats and cheeses. It never occurred to me that those items were dead animals. I'm not sure at what age I learned the facts, but I do remember that it was talked and joked about as normal and necessary. It was the slow conditioning that most of us experienced. It was the acceptable norm. When I think back, I did see trucks full of cows and pigs often, but in my mind I thought they were being moved to another farm for some reason.

My mind never entered the slaughterhouse until later.

My grandparents were raised on Iowa farms. For them, the business of animals for food was survival—actually, not only for them, but for Iowa itself. It was the major industry besides corn and insurance. Eating meat and potatoes every day was your birthright in Iowa; for some this still remains true. It goes so deep that many people fight hard against the idea of veganism. It's like you are trying to strip them of their name or something very dear to their identity.

Food was always a huge part of our family celebrations as it is for most people. Both of my grandmothers cooked for the family for all holidays and birthdays. Some occasions, we would have a ham and a turkey. Meat was always the main course, and there was more than enough for everyone. In fact, at times it seemed the goal was to eat ourselves to sleep and then lay around like walrus. I have many happy memories, and it's not so much about the food but more about the people. However, food ties us to our families and to the memories. I don't eat meat now, but I would never give up my grandma's vegetable casserole or apple salad. I had to modify them a bit, but I just consider that as modernizing the dishes. Sometimes I say I modernize, and sometimes I say I veganize. For me, it means the same thing.

When I first became vegetarian as an adult in Iowa, people would call me odd and were very closed off to the idea. When I went to parties, I would eat mustard on a bun often. No one was trying to accommodate this strange diet that I had chosen. Back then, I lived on noodles and bread. It's a good thing I was young because it didn't affect me badly at all. That was my diet for years, and I rarely ate fruit and a small amount of vegetables. It really was noodles, noodles, and more noodles. My friends would say "All Deanna eats are noodles all day long." It was true, and I weighed 110 pounds. Ah, the good ol' days when I existed on coffee, cigarettes, noodles, and grunge music. It was the '90s and I was definitely not a health nut; but I did love animals, so that led me to vegetarianism.

I was born an Iowa girl and there is still some Iowa in me for sure, but I have always been very open-minded and curious. I have taken this Iowan around the world and into the realm of new ideas. It's been quite a ride so far and this is only the beginning.

My Road to Veganism

It wasn't Perfect but it's Mine

My road to veganism was bumpy and imperfect, but I am not ashamed of stumbling and making mistakes in life. Ultimately, all the details, good and bad, brought me here to a place of contentment and passion in my vegan life. Being honest and striving to improve is of importance to me.

My introduction to eating organic and vegetarian was in my childhood from around eleven to fourteen years old. My mom married my Italian stepdad Alfredo, aka Fred, and he was very into gardening and canning food. I remember lots of sprouts, even in the brownies. We had food all year round from our garden, canned in the basement. My dad and my grandparents had huge gardens as well, so I was always around fresh and good quality vegetables. I mostly complained about vegetables back then and wanted to eat McDonald's, chips, and pizza like all my friends did. I enjoyed the tomatoes and hot peppers but that was about it. I see now what an incredible effort it was to grow food and prepare such quality meals.

At age fourteen, I was struggling and very unhappy in my home life, so I moved in with my maternal grandparents. Living with my grandma and grandpa for those few years was really good for me, and I am still grateful for it. My grandma Mildred catered to me and made most of my meals, almost all of which contained meat and dairy. She was an amazing cook and I loved it. I had ice cream almost every night for a snack. My meals at that time were very Iowa, Midwestern fare. My grandmother did make lots of veggies and fruit salads as well, but sometimes even those contained dairy. Enjoying big elaborate dinners was part of my childhood on both sides of my family and we did eat a wide variety of food. Since gardening was big on both sides, luckily the veggies were high quality and organic, not what you find at some mainstream grocery stores today. It's a shame that unless you go organic or the farmer's market route, you may get petrified rocks with no flavor these days. I do understand why some people say they hate vegetables. If they are low quality, they taste like nothing.

When I was nineteen, I had what I call my religious experience with a cow and I stopped eating meat for many years. I was at a stoplight behind a semi full of cows, waiting to turn left. There was this one cow staring right at me with those big brown eyes. I started to feel shaky and anxiety-ridden. I felt trapped and fearful but I couldn't look away. I just knew it was how the animal felt, and somehow I was feeling it. It was the longest red light and time stood still. Finally, the light turned green and it was as though a lengthy and thought-out communication had happened. I know it sounds crazy, but I gave up meat that moment. It was easy after that experience. I still think about that one particular cow that was able to reach me and have such an impact on my life. I rarely brought it up right after it happened because I knew what people would think, but anyone who knows me well has heard about it. Now, after all these years, it means even more to me; it was significant and special. I have amazing experiences with animals often, but not like that. That day was mind-blowing and it changed me.

Giving up meat was not difficult for me, but I would go in and out of eating cheese and eggs. Sometimes I would give it up and then I would eat it for a while again. I was very wishy-washy about dairy. I had no idea at that time how cruel the dairy business was to animals, so I was in the dark as many people are to this day.

After years of no animal flesh, my train went off the tracks, and I feel I must share what happened during that time. Around 1998, I was at a friend's Thanksgiving dinner and I ate a few bites of turkey for the first time in years. I don't know what possessed me to do that. After that night, I was eating meat again for about three years without much thought. Not to the level of the average American, by any means, but at all was strange for me, after being vegetarian for years. I was struggling with my demons at that time. I was very self-destructive in many ways. It was one of the ways I really dishonored myself and my beliefs.

I met my future husband Kevin in 2000, working at Guido's, an Italian restaurant in Santa Monica, but we didn't start dating until 2001. When I first met him, I thought he was a wonderful guy but too nice for me. He thought I was, in his words, "kind of bitchy." That is very general if you ask me, and I just think I am very assertive. I speak my mind and I am not a pushover. Still he tried to kiss me and even playfully kidnapped me one night by hopping on the freeway instead of turning on my street when giving me a ride home. He took me to a party and told everyone I was his fiancée. I barely knew him. On the way home he sang '70s rock songs at the top of his lungs. That part I kind of liked, but I thought he was nuts too. After that night, I wrote him off as just a wacky guy, and he left Guido's and went to work at James Beach. A good year went by and he ended up coming back to Guido's. The moment he walked in, I turned around and he looked entirely different to me. Love at second sight.

From that eve on, we were inseparable. I felt very comfortable around him and I could totally be myself. Basically, we could be weird together and that's the best.

Kevin had the worst eating habits of anyone I had ever met. One day, he drove through Weinerschnitzel and ordered five cheeseburgers. I was blown away. I think his over-the-top bad habits sparked something in me that started me on the path back to vegetarianism and ultimately to veganism. He had this American fast food way of life that I definitely didn't enjoy witnessing.

We were party animals at that time. I had a group of friends that I ran with called the fourth street players. We gave ourselves that name. There was the General, and one of my nicknames was Detroit, and a bunch of other nuts joined together at the hip. That was a really outlandishly fun time in my life because we were like a crazy family. I did drink too much. After awhile, my little family started to break up as a few moved away from LA and a few turned out not being lifelong-friend material. This was probably a good thing and for the best. I had Kevin through the transition and we were in love and got engaged very quickly, after only six months together.

One of our hobbies was going out to eat, and I started thinking about vegetarianism again and the animals. It got to the point that I would go out to eat and then come home and cry about it like a lunatic. How could I, of all people, eat animals? I was vegetarian for so many years.

I had let myself get so disconnected from animals in general, but this all changed when we adopted a little dog we named Georgia. She was my first dog as an adult, and I had no idea the profound effect she would have on me. She was so attuned to my moods and feelings. Our connection was and still is strong. She woke me up from my hazy phase, and I started to see again. I am so thankful for Georgia because like the cow years before, she was able to reach me. I would spend time with her and bond with her and it made me realize once again that each animal is an individual.

There were other factors, good and bad, but the point is that my conscience woke up and with a vengeance. I became vegetarian again, which made me really perk up, but it wasn't enough. I now had guilt that I knew better and went against it. I started to really look at myself, and that wasn't easy. I had always admired people of strong conviction. I was one of those people until I lost my way. I had tremendous regard for David Merrill, the director whose story was told in the film *Guilty by Suspicion*, and I was also set on fire by the movie *JFK*, mostly because I loved Jim Garrison's pursuit of the truth. The way Oliver Stone depicted it made me want to know every detail as he did. Somewhere along the way, I had lost my conviction and my truth about a lot of things and I desperately wanted it back.

I decided to become vegan. There were some months of transitioning. My last two things were cheese and sushi. The two things I could not imagine living without. I wasn't even really a vegetarian. Technically, I was a lacto pescatarian or something like that. I was a sushi addict for many years, and not the rolls, but yellowtail sashimi was my favorite.

I looked at fish as totally separate from animals until I watched how they were killed. Some of them were so big, bigger than I imagined, and they were flopping around furiously and looked like they were in terrible pain. That was it for me. Cheese was also a constant until I learned about the horrible animal cruelty, and now I abhor the idea of dairy cheese. I was determined to go all the way and walk the walk.

I am a huge animal lover and when I am open, I have an incredible connection to them. It was time for me to go all the way and with conviction. I made this choice and I didn't look back. It was by far one of the best decisions I have made in this life. It has changed me in every way. It encompasses so much that is difficult to understand until you live it. I hope everyone gets this chance.

I'll just tell you what it did for and to me. First of all I devoured every book, film, or clip I could get my hot little hands on for several years regarding food and nutrition, animals used for food, entertainment and clothing, and the impact on the environment. I learned so much and with each new bit of information, my resolve grew stronger. I am so vegan now that it should be my middle name. Seeing those animals being tortured and disrespected made it impossible to be anything else. I view undercover animal activists as the most incredible people. Those videos are heartbreaking to watch, but I made myself watch most multiple times. If the animals had to endure that torture only to be murdered, the least I could do is open my eyes and see it. I wanted to grow and I wanted to improve and sometimes that is not easy or pleasant. Harder than watching the videos was realizing the hypocrite I had become. I no longer wanted to be the animal lover who also ate animals. In fact, I wanted to be the animal lover who fought to protect and help them, and to do that, I had to see the hardcore truth.

Another benefit of veganism for me is that I used to suffer horribly from depression. I suppose it's possible that it was a coincidence, but going vegan lifted a lot of that. After years of very dark depressive periods, I don't suffer like that any longer. I feel lighter in every way, physically, emotionally, and most of all, spiritually. Do I still have bad days here and there and some depression? Of course I do, but for anyone who has battled real depression and extreme ups and downs, you know it's another level. It's the deepest, darkest black hole and when you are in it, you cannot see a way out. I used to call it my cocoon and then I would emerge a butterfly eventually, happy again. I can't explain it but after going vegan, this started to diminish and now it is not so much a constant part of my reality. There are contributing factors for certain, but I believe that veganism has helped me in that area.

I am a loner and I don't like labels. It's difficult for me to be a group person or to be associated long-term with groups, but I *am vegan*. I am proud to call myself vegan all day long. For me it stands for justice, love of animals, and conviction.

Well, that is the condensed version of my imperfect road to veganism. For each person, it will be a unique tale. One is not better than the other, just different. I mean it when I say I hope every person gets this amazing opportunity. It will open you up and change the way you look at life. That is what it has done for me.

Nonvegan Family and Friends

Find the positive and diffuse the negative

I see many vegans and especially aspiring vegans suffer in this area. They so badly want to be supported and understood in their choices. For some vegans the support and caring is there, but for many it is not. It's important to remember that being vegan goes against what most of us were taught and how we were raised. Change is not easy for many folks. I personally thrive on change, but I don't think that is the case for many people.

I have had years of experience living vegan and dealing with my family and friends, and the reactions have varied considerably. I have been very supported, and even some family members and friends are now vegan as well. I have also lost a few friends over living vegan. You might think it was my choice but on the contrary, the friends I have lost have been the ones who could not come to terms with me not eating animals any longer. I am referring to the friends who were continually rude and angry about it. The ones who never missed an opportunity to slam anything about being vegetarian or vegan. I know now that losing such friendships was destined to happen over something. Some people's beliefs are very rigid and immovable. I have many friends who still eat meat. Do I wish they didn't? Of course, but they have to come to this decision on their own, as I did. I can inspire and help, but being rude and forceful rarely works, no matter which side of the issue you are on.

I have had heated debates with many people over this topic. I have told people off big-time online and in person. I am not proud of it but it has happened. I have a temper and the lion has roared. Today I strive to be a good example of living vegan happily and very healthily and not to preach or judge. Still I am human, and honestly, I like to debate intelligently. I want to go on record and say that when people go off on a tangent and start insulting me, I will fight back, and at times it has not been pretty. It's not my favorite thing about myself but I am working on it. I do think I have improved regarding veganism. I do ask that if you are going to debate this important topic, please come up with something beyond your opinion, based on conditioning and silly statements like "I like bacon" and "Don't we need the protein?" Animals suffer greatly and people suffer with many health issues as a result of choosing to eat animals, so my hope is that people will grow to take this more seriously as a society.

I have done my research, so lots of times a few facts and figures will shut up the harshest critics. In my opinion, some people are a lost cause and I won't waste much time discussing it with them. The good news is that an incredible amount of people just don't know a lot about it but are open to learning. I get lots of emails and messages from people asking general questions and also telling me that they are starting to live vegan. This is what makes me so happy. I love these messages and I could never get too many of them. I will go out of my way to help anyone trying to go vegan.

One thing that I think is very important to gain acceptance from your close personals when doing anything, being vegan included, is to have conviction. When and if you waiver, they will pounce. I am not saying you have to live as this perfect little angel who never makes a mistake, but if you are in the process of being vegan but not quite there, I would not preach about it. It's important to be authentic and honest with yourself and others about where you are in the process. It's never about being this perfect person. It's about making better choices for yourself, your loved ones, animals, and the earth. Each step to more thoughtful choices and informed living is amazing and should be celebrated. In the beginning, I mostly celebrated my little victories with my dog Georgia and my husband.

I found it invigorating when I would learn something new or discover a negative that I wasn't going to support any longer. I felt like yelling "I'm in charge now."

Finally, I started to feel freedom from advertising and corporations. I had lifted the big curtain and I saw Oz with my own eyes. It was cool, and I still have those moments because there is always more to learn and discover. Additionally, we have to keep a watchful eye because there are those greedy people who will choose money above all else, even if it means people and animals suffer. This is the number one reason it is important to be awake and aware.

My focus is to keep it positive and keep improving my knowledge and decisions. Do I always succeed everyday in this? No, but I already covered that, so I just keep it moving forward.

My advice, in a nutshell, is to surround yourself with supportive people. Regarding the unsupportive people, you need to be direct and let them know you are trying to improve, and don't appreciate their negativity. Keep going, learning, and growing.

How One Affects the Other

One question I get asked often is "How did you get your husband to become vegan?" The easy answer is that I didn't. He has a mind of his own. I certainly had some influence on him, but you cannot force things on people you love. I talked to him about it quite a bit, showed him a few films, and introduced him to books. Luckily, he has an open mind and a heart for animals. I have watched him grow from the guy who ordered five cheeseburgers at the drive-through and said our first puppy could not sleep in the bed to the man who is a doting doggy dad and animal rescuer. It's been so cool to witness the growth. Over the years, he has waivered a bit and had a slice of cheese pizza here and there, but overall, the change is pretty amazing. Sometimes I have to tell him to tone it down because he gets so passionate telling people about the horrible hell the animals go through in slaughterhouses. I believe that in all of us is a knowing that treating animals with such disrespect and cruelty is wrong, except maybe in serial killers. They are known to enjoy torturing animals for fun. This is a very small percentage of folks. It is so easy for people to disconnect from the animals killed for food and their suffering because someone else does the dirty work, and people simply go to a store and pick up the packaged meat.

ONE VEGAN MAMA

I became vegan because of my love and respect for animals. My husband and I are opposites in many ways, but at least we can agree on compassion for animals and others in general. It's a pretty cool thing to bond on and share with your significant other. It ends up spilling into so many other areas. For instance, we have rescued many dogs, cats, birds, and even helped a bear get relocated from a small cage to a sprawling sanctuary. Our dogs are our other three kids and help make our lives richer. We love teaching our daughter about protecting animals and eating with a conscience. Cooking at home and going out to eat are intense hobbies for us, and we love trying new recipes and restaurants. All in all, sharing this worldview of veganism bonds us as a family in endless ways.

I do realize that it can be difficult when one partner is vegan and the other isn't. Some people can manage it and be harmonious, but I am sure it isn't easy. At this point in my life, meat in my fridge might as well be a dead dog or cat because I view it the same way. I cannot have any dead animals in my refrigerator.

Once the conditioning is broken, it changes not only one's thinking but also what looks and smells good or offensive. I used to live on sushi, and now, when I smell dead fish, it almost gags me. I guess it could be compared to a smoker versus a nonsmoker. Not that this applies to me any longer, but I cannot imagine kissing someone after they had a steak. I'd rather lick the pavement. I bet single vegans feel this, and it is yet another big consideration about compatibility.

When people barbecue animals, the smell is so gross to me and it gets in my hair. I am not that in to my hair smelling like a dead and cooked animal. Some people think vegans are depriving themselves, when in fact, meat and dairy make me think of old garbage and I immediately envision what the animals suffered. Not to mention I know how dirty and bacteria ridden those places (slaughterhouses) are, and lastly, I remember all the drugs (antibiotics and hormones) that go into the animals. I am not depriving myself. I just don't care for that stuff. I am happy my significant other feels the same; otherwise, his eating habits could torment me daily.

One of the major things that eventually come to the forefront in relationships is how we take care of ourselves. The goal for most is to have a long, happy, and healthy life together, accomplishing things and having adventures. It's quite helpful if both people stay at a decent weight and don't cause themselves multiple unnecessary health issues.

Don't get me wrong, some health issues are somewhat unavoidable. However, I think we can all agree that what one eats contributes to weight issues and unwanted ailments and disease. It is beneficial if both people at least try to stay healthy. Of course we will all have sickness and unwanted health concerns as we age, but eating well can drastically minimize that.

Food is such a central thing in all of our lives, so of course, it plays a big role in all relationships. We need it to live, but for many, it can be addiction. I do think I was addicted to cheese. I used to eat it daily, and I would practically knock someone over to get that last slice of Gouda on the hors d'oeuvres plate. Now, no, thank you. It's good to keep our food addictions and obsessions in balance. I will admit I still struggle with not devouring all the vegan cheese in the house in one day. It's a constant work in progress. If people would cut down on their meat consumption, the demand would not be as great, so less animals would be crammed into these buildings, which equals less suffering, less drugs needed, less disease, and less impact on our planet. Ideally we would support one another in improving our daily choices.

Families and couples support each other in the good and the bad habits and addictions. Smokers tend to be around other smokers. Drug addicts can be found most times around other drug addicts. Meat eaters can be found at the steakhouses and vegans at the vegan restaurants. All that is a no-brainer. Sure, there are random groups of mixed company all the time, but similar interests and ways of living create connection. However, what many don't think about is that at some point, each person made a decision or didn't and let someone else make it for them.

I took a morals and ethics class in college many years ago. One thing the professor said has always stuck in my head: "Decide who you are before you go to the party." Decide you are *not* a cocaine user, so when it is presented, you have already made your decision; therefore, you just say, "No, that's not my thing." If you are on the fence, chances are you will be easily convinced to follow along with the others. The thing about meat and dairy is that when it was first given to you, drugs and all, you were most likely a small child, so the decision was essentially made for you, not by you. What if you had been given all the facts and a choice as a child? Would your decision to eat meat have been the same?

That brings me to our relationship with our grandparents and parents regarding food. In most cases, they made incredible effort to feed us well. I am sure it is perplexing to many of them when they hear about veganism. When my grandparents were growing up, there was no such thing as a factory farm, not to their knowledge anyway. Animals primarily lived on real farms with grass, but that is not the case today. They were not shot up with hormones or antibiotics. It was extremely different. It was in my parents' childhood that fast food and processing animals as things—not beings—went into overdrive. It was sold to the general public as convenience. The way the animals were being objectified was not shown, just the fact that you could get a burger, fries, and a soda at the diner and pretty quickly. It makes sense that we would have a somewhat different relationship to food than our grandparents and parents because things have changed drastically. Now we have to worry about all the drugs and hormones, the GMOs, and the latest is that chickens will be sent to China alive and then sent back to the USA and sold as food. Everyone should be worried about that one. Not to mention the number of animals crammed and tortured in these big industrial buildings has grown to a "beyond any shred of decency" level. It is up to us to demand better for the animals and our own health.

The last relationship mentioned or thought about is the one between the workers in these slaughterhouses and the animals. I've viewed an incredible amount of undercover footage.

There are some slaughterhouse workers who are going through the motions in a disconnected way, a defense mechanism perhaps to a very undesirable job. Then you have the real "sick in the head" men who I witnessed laughing and enjoying hurting the animals. The footage I saw at one Hormel plant in Iowa a couple years ago was beyond what I could have imagined. They were sticking metal rods up the pig's butts for fun. It was heartbreaking and unbelievable. It's scary to me that some of these men roam free in our world. Do you think these are well-adjusted people? I am sure some people enter this job somewhat sane. Do you think after killing hundreds or thousands of animals daily— while they scream, blood everywhere, the smell, the sounds, their eyes, the desperation and the fear all around—that these men remain mentally stable? Would you be able to do that job for a month and feel good and happy? There is a book called *Slaughterhouse* by Gail Eisnitz; several previous workers were interviewed, and their experiences sound like hell on earth, if you ask me. It is our responsibility to ask the hard questions because these workers are doing the dirty work for meat and dairy consumers. They are killing animals every day for you (meat eaters). The consumer is paying for this entire process. It always amazes me how people don't want to hear about the abuse of the animals, but they are paying for it. If it is too terrible for you to hear about, perhaps it should be too terrible for you to pay to have it done.

Depending on your upbringing, geographic location, family, friends, and significant other, you have a certain way of looking at food. It's not a bad idea to ponder this and ask yourself some questions about your choices and the choices made for you by someone else. The decisions you make or don't make are affecting you, people around you, animals, and the very planet we live on every day.

My Vegan Pregnancy

Life is an Adventure Full of Twists and Turns

My husband and I talked about kids before we got married, and we were both open to having babies, but I also had a dream of adopting and he was agreeable to that. I read an article about Chinese girls getting left on orphanage steps and in parks, and that planted in my mind the idea of adopting a baby girl from China. Later, I realized how many children there were right here in my own city in need of a home and love. If I do adopt in the future, I cannot say for sure where the child will be from but I have a feeling I won't have to look very far.

After getting married twice (once secretly in Vegas and then again a year later for family and friends) to the same man, about five years went by without much more than a fleeting thought or joking remark about having a baby or adopting. We were having too much fun traveling and just living life at Venice Beach. Not to mention that I wasn't entirely sure I even wanted to be a mom. It was a big maybe. I wanted to be positive that I had something to offer. So many kids are brought into the world on a whim, and I wanted to be prepared.

We started to get our act together and bought a couple houses, one for investment and one to live in. My husband brought it up that he still had the hope of a biological child, so after many conversations, we agreed it was a great time to try. I was a really dedicated mom to my three pooches and we were pretty settled and in a good place. I thought it would happen immediately even though I had been on the pill for my entire adult life. Every month I was shocked that I was not with child. After months of no luck, I went on Google about getting pregnant and read that counting your ovulation could help. So the next month, I counted twelve days from the first day of my period and made sure we were creating magic in the bedroom on the twelfth and many days after that, and bam! I was pregnant that month, piece of cake. I was so thrilled and felt amazing. I didn't have morning sickness at all and I was just so happy. I think it took me getting pregnant to realize how much I wanted a baby. I was over the moon and planning like crazy.

I was around seven or eight weeks along. I just knew it was a girl although it wasn't time to find out. I had a serious sweet tooth, so one day I ran to the Whole Foods for a cupcake. I brought it home and was watching Oprah. Out of the blue, I started feeling these cramps so I ran to the bathroom and there was blood. I started to cry and beg, "Oh God, please don't take my baby." I am not super religious but I am spiritual. I do believe in something larger than myself and this life. I started to try to bargain. I'll give this up and do that if you just don't take my baby. The bleeding became heavier, and I drove myself to the hospital. I called my husband on the way there and he left work to meet me. The rest is a blur except for the part where the doctor said miscarriage. All I could think was that my baby died and *why*? I just lay there in shock, with this stabbing pain in my heart. All I wanted to do was go home and cry, but I had to wait for a shot called Rogam because I am blood type O negative and it is necessary for future pregnancies to go full-term. By the time my husband arrived, I was just a shell there in the hospital bed. That was one of my worst days. Even now, when I hear of a woman miscarrying, I am transported back to that day and I feel a connection of heartbreak and loss. I had no idea how common miscarriage was until it happened to me because people don't talk about it enough.

I can really torment myself, and I definitely did during this time. My husband stayed positive and said "We will have our child, you'll see." During this time, I talked my husband into getting foster and adoption certified. We took classes and learned a lot. We did what is called respite care for three children. Basically, the child is in between their birth home and a foster but the decisions have not been made yet.

The first one was a wonderful seven-year-old boy. His mother had made some bad choices in the boyfriend department and he was taken away. She was trying to make the necessary changes and get her son back. In the meantime, he stayed with us. He was used to fast food and lots of meat, so I wondered how he would transition; but to my surprise, he loved our vegan food. One eve, he said, "These nuggets are better than the other ones," referring to the faux nuggets made of tofu at one of our favorite restaurants, Vinh Loi Tofu. I had so much fun taking him to the library and to see the horses.

He was a joy, but I was glad when he was reunited with his mother. I felt like we helped a family.

Next was a two-and-a-half-year-old boy of a well-known father. Both parents were going through personal struggles. I think I became the most attached to him and he to me because of his age. We had him for a short time, but I adored him and I am glad I could be there for him. He ended up living with his grandmother. She was thoughtful and even called me a few times, but it was best to let them move on from a difficult time without me to remind them. It was okay that he wouldn't remember me. I will remember him, and I'm glad it was me who got the call. It was plain to see how loved he was by his parents and family. I think it would be impossible not to fall in love with a little two- and-a-half-year-old put into such a vulnerable position.

The third child we had in our home was a ten-year-old boy who had the saddest story. He was terribly abused by his mother and would not be going back to her. He had been shuffled around from foster home to foster home. He needed a place to stay while decisions were made about the next steps for him. I found out he had a fascination with cooking but was not allowed in the kitchen, so he and I would cook dinner together. He put a pinch of sugar in everything. It was pretty funny and surprisingly good. I told him he would probably grow up to be a chef. He went into a residential home to have therapy and other care. I have kept tabs on him.

After close to a year, I decided to see an expert to make sure we were doing all we could for a biological child. I decided to try only three more months, and if no pregnancy happened, we would adopt. My heart just couldn't take more than three months. I said I would do the ovulation pills and the shot to stimulate ovulation, but not IVF. If it was meant to be, this baby had three months. My doctor advised that longer would be better, but I said no! I was ready to be a mom so a long-drawn-out thing wasn't for me, and I already loved the idea of adoption. The first month, I got pregnant. Sadly, as quick as it came, it left. They call it a chemical pregnancy. To me, it was another loss. The next month, nothing, except good ol' Aunt Flow and I were not optimistic. The third and final month was approaching, and I was driving home from the doctor and these two names together came to me—Ever Olivia. I actually said out loud, "Wow, that's pretty. If you want that to be your name, now is the time." On the third month, to my amazement, I got pregnant. Everything went smoothly, and the most incredible person came into my life. The minute I saw her, I felt that I had been waiting for her to arrive my entire life. This is strange because I said for ages that I wasn't sure about marriage or kids. I was so independent and didn't see myself as maternal. I was so wrong.

It's funny the amount of things I have been wrong about. I also enjoyed being pregnant. My husband says it was the happiest he has ever seen me. I was the glowing and giddy pregnant one, and women were so kind to me during that time. I found that nice but puzzling. My hormones had me giggling and smiling all the time.

Many people asked me about being vegan while pregnant. I first started thinking of this book at that time. I realized that there was such a curiosity and interest in my pregnancy. I could tell that some thought it was the wrong choice. I knew it was the only choice for me, and I did my research. My doctor was very supportive and never questioned my choice to be vegan while pregnant. We discussed it and he said, "You have been vegan for years and you are very healthy." I also received many messages from vegetarian and vegan women asking me questions and commending my choice. It didn't really occur to me that I was doing something so different until all the questions started to become frequent.

Some people actually said to me that I would crave meat while pregnant. Why would I? I hadn't eaten it in years. I'll tell you what I craved most—green apples and potatoes. I ate bags and bags of green apples, more in nine months than in the previous ten years. I have never been a potato person but I sure was during pregnancy. Any sort of potato I would eat in massive quantities. Not one craving for meat. I did devour a few veggie burgers, lots of tofu scrambles, veggie and bean soups, and just a ton of different veggies and fruits.

I took prenatal vitamins prior to and during my pregnancy. I made sure to eat a wide variety of food and did yoga. I had the most awesome pregnancy and truly enjoyed it. I would highly recommend a vegan pregnancy.

I gained twenty-five pounds total. I still felt like a whale at the end and was ready to pop. That last month is a long one, as every pregnant lady knows.

I was back to my prepregnancy weight in about eight weeks and posing in a bikini by month six. Don't get me wrong, I had to get on the treadmill and work hard for those last few pounds, but I believe being vegan helped me overall.

My daughter was born with eyes wide open, ready for her place in this crazy world. She's healthy, thriving, and smart, and not one animal had to die for her to be her best. I look at her and think, *She is the hope for a more compassionate future.* Her and all the other vegan babies.

My Vegan Toddler

She is Happy, Healthy, and Thriving

Many mothers ask me so earnestly, "What does she eat?" The list is quite long of what she does eat, so I usually just say she eats everything except meat and dairy. She is now three, and her openness to try new things is expanding again. For a time, it was somewhat limited because *no* was her favorite word, and she enjoyed using it.

I'll give you a quick rundown of some things she loves right now. She likes farfalle pasta, which she calls bows. I make quinoa pasta because it's higher in protein, and I use olive oil and nutritional yeast flakes on all of her pasta dishes. If you haven't noticed yet, we love nutritional yeast flakes around here. She goes crazy for most fruit, especially mangoes and strawberries. She loves tofu scrambles with peas, faux chicken nuggets with sweet potato fries, and veggie burgers with a plain bun. Every Saturday and Sunday, she makes pancakes with her daddy. You can find the vegan mix at Wholefoods or Sprouts. She snacks on seaweed crisps, carrots, bananas, cookies, chips, apples, soy yogurt, popsicles, cupcakes, crackers, almond ice cream, and so many other things. She absolutely loves smoothies, and vanilla is her favorite flavor. I use PlantFusion protein powder, banana, almond or peanut butter, almond or soymilk, hempseeds, dates, and ice. I also sneak a little spinach or arugula in there too.

When she is not eating her vegetables very well, I use this powder called Kidz SuperFood by Amazing Grass. One scoop is three servings of fruits and veggies. I put it in her juice. I also put flaxseed oil in her juice for omega-3s sometimes.

She drinks soymilk and almond milk, water, and juice for beverages. She takes a multivitamin, and we switch that up. She eats a wide variety of food and gets more protein than the recommended daily amount. She is a healthy child, and her immunity is excellent because we don't deal with her being constantly sick, as I see some people go through with their kids, and she is around sick kids at preschool.

One challenging aspect about having a vegan toddler is the kid party circuit, which is Chuck E. Cheese's pizza parties and dairy-made cupcakes and such. Some people surprise me and have options for her like vegan cupcakes and vegan cheese on the pizza. I love that. Thank you to those considerate and aware parents. In general, I call and ask if this is an issue, and if they seem put out, I simply bring a vegan slice of pizza and a few vegan cupcakes.

At preschool, they do make things nonvegan, treats such as Jell-O and cookies with dairy, so I just bring a vegan alternative. At this point, my daughter does somewhat understand that we don't eat some things that others do. She knows it has to do with kindness to animals. At age three, that is all she needs to understand,

and I fill in the blanks with similar food items when necessary. Each year as she grows, I will explain a bit more. We do eat very healthy, but she also gets the typical kid foods like burgers, pizza, chips, cupcakes, popcorn, and so on occasionally, but hers are not made with any animal products. She loves animals as most children do, and I don't want to feed them to her without her knowledge.

Even in California, we are still the minority in many situations, but we are happy, and I am confident things are coming along. Big changes are on the horizon. It takes confidence and strength to do what you know is right even if the majority isn't quite there.

My daughter's opinions and preferences are important to me. I know she will have many questions not just about veganism but all of my choices, and I will answer them as they are presented. In the meantime, I love teaching her about respecting others, including animals, and being kind.

The Traveling Vegan

A little preparation goes a long way

My husband and I bonded on our love of roaming around this big and interesting planet. I would go almost anywhere once just to see it. I love visiting other countries, and I love road tripping around my own. Whether I am going to Italy or Iowa, I can veganize the whole trip, no problem. I have been doing it for a long time, so I've had practice.

Snacks

I do nuts and dried fruit combos in pouches and small Tupperware containers for quick snacks. I love Tofurky Jurky and order a box before an overseas trip. It's easy and tasty for long trips. Travel-size soymilk is a staple for my toddler, and a little dark chocolate never hurt anyone. I eat dried peas with sea salt or kale chips for an alternative to potato chips. It only takes a few minutes to think ahead and bring healthy and tasty treats instead of depending on gas stations and fast food joints. Things are improving, but we cannot count on healthy snacks being available everywhere yet.

Breakfast

Many people ask me what in the heck I eat for breakfast, and it seems in travel this could be even more perplexing.

Get ready because this will blow your mind—coffee and a banana. I am not a big breakfast person. I know many people are, so I take notice what is offered at the continental breakfast in hotels. It's easy; there's the toast or a bagel with peanut butter. Potatoes and hash browns are usually available. Fruit is all vegan all the time, and most spreads offer oatmeal.

My daughter likes cereal with one of the travel soymilk boxes and toast with peanut butter only. My husband will get a little of everything.

Many cities and towns have vegetarian and vegan restaurants now, so check with the hotel or the VegOut app on smartphones for local spots, and you might get an amazing vegan breakfast that will surprise you.

Lunch

We like to stop and have a nice lunch. I check for vegan places, and I am happy to say many times there are a few. This wasn't the case ten years ago, and that is so exciting.

If we end up at a chain restaurant or local spot, I check the appetizers and sides to see if I can create a unique vegan plate. I also ask what seasonal veggies they have in stock and how they can be prepared.

For fast food, I recommend Burger King for the veggie burger, or one of the Mexican chains for a veggie burrito, minus the cheese, plus extra avocado.

Dinner

I love dressing up and eating out. It's an intense hobby, and I am pretty good at it. I like to reinvent my look and try new foods when I get away. I travel to expand. I don't want it to be anything like home; otherwise why wouldn't I just stay home? The first thing I do is look for a vegan or veg- friendly place and if I cannot find that, I will look for ethnic, like Indian, Ethiopian, Mexican, or Italian. Obviously if I am in Italy or Mexico, I will choose accordingly. When in Rome, I have a lot of Minestrone soup, bread, spaghetti with green olives, and lots of red wine. That does it for me.

Your selections might be different, but once you get into thinking vegan you will see that it is endless.

I am not much of a camper, but I do love to grill out. I am from Iowa after all. We have a huge grill and probably fire it up more than the average carnivore. If I were to go camping, I would do epic veggie burgers with all the condiments and onions, mushrooms, tomatoes, and pickles, maybe vegan cheese too. I would do grilled Portobello mushrooms and veggie skewers. I also love to do avocado on the grill, green beans in tinfoil with onions and garlic and Field Roast vegan sausages.

The bottom line is that vegans eat everything in travel that they do at home. We eat many things that you do, with the exclusion of the dead animals and other species milk.

If you really stop and contemplate it, you might understand. I don't want to drink a cow's milk anymore than I want to drink milk from some woman's boob or the nursing cat down the block. I would just rather not.

Vegan can work anywhere. Here is the best tip I can offer. Order and eat anything they have available except the meat and dairy. You can create your own plate. A steamed or roasted veggie plate, or a pasta dish, is easy. If you are doing low carb, ask for more veggies and sauce than noodles. If they offer pizza, ask for it without cheese. I have been disappointed a few times but also had some of my best pizzas this way. Let's get real; there is always a chance of disappointment at any restaurant. I have noticed that when with a group, I am pleased with my selection more than the average person.

Traveling vegan is not difficult. It's just a choice like everything else. I enjoy seeing which places are going vegan fastest and which ones are far behind. It's very interesting. For example, Portland, Oregon, is amazing. It's like vegan land. Many Southern and Midwestern places are truly lacking, but I see surprising glimpses of change. On my last trip to Des Moines, Iowa, a pizza place was advertising vegan pizza on the radio. I thought I was hearing things but it was true.

Believe it or not, vegan is coming to your town. No matter where you roam, you will find animal lovers, compassionate souls, and people who care for the planet and the health of humans. These people are referred to positively, sometimes negatively, and happily call themselves vegans. Traveling vegan can be a challenge, depending on where you go and how you get there, but this is improving quickly.

Future Fashion

Compassion is the most beautiful fashion

This is a very important topic if you ask me. I have always enjoyed fashion. For me it's total fun. I like to go high-end, vintage, and inexpensive for any fleeting trends. I may be a devoted vegan but this does not slow me down in the fashion department one bit. It has actually helped me to define my style. I am a hat girl. I have about seventy-five hats and counting. A hat and a pair of chic sunglasses make me feel glamorous even if I am wearing jeans and a tank top.

I still brake for shoes and handbags like a lunatic. I am a woman after all. I just ask if they are leather or not. The sales ladies usually think I want them to be leather, so that gives me a chance to explain why I choose nonleather.

I used to carry Coach, Louis Vuitton, and Lamb, to name a few of my past favorites. I would spare no expense and I am embarrassed to say that I spent $700 on a pair of leather shoes once. I was a total sucker for the name on the inside that no one would ever see. I am mostly ashamed that animals gave their lives for my fashion whimsy.

Our style can be such a creative statement about us, but it can also just as easily be a moral statement, and a powerful one. It can say so much about who we are and what we believe in.

Leather is a dirty word to me now. No leather seats in my car and absolutely no leather handbags or shoes. I would not enjoy a dead and quite-sticky leather couch either. No, thank you. Becoming vegan freed me from being a slave to brand names and opened me up to buy ethically and also what I really like. I definitely feel that I have my own personal style instead of a keeping up with the Joneses' wardrobe. The funny thing is that I get more compliments now than I ever did on the Louis Vuittons and such. I get asked about my purses, and many times I am carrying Susan Nichole handbags. They are my absolute favorite, and I collect them.

If you are a label diva and cannot imagine not flaunting the haute couture names, then Stella McCartney items are equally expensive and prestigious but are ethically made, no animal skins. You can spend a ton of money if you need to on vegan items as well, so knock yourself out. I do love her clothes and shoes with a passion, but I only possess a couple Stella McCartney items. You can be styled out and still be thoughtful about what you purchase. I love discovering new designers as well as being loyal to great designers like Susan Nichole and Matt & Nat. For shoes, I look everywhere because many designers make nonleather shoes now and they are half the price of the others. I buy a few pairs at a time instead of one. For instance Chinese Laundry has some leather and some nonleather shoes, and lots of companies do. You just need to check the labels and ask. The more nonleather that is purchased, the cuter these less expensive and cruelty-free items will become, and this is good for us and the animals. Do you have any idea how fun it is to buy three pairs of shoes guilt-free? Well, I do, and I used to get buyer's remorse over one pair of leather shoes. Fur is just plain disgusting, in my opinion. For those who still wear it, I have only these words: it's a fashion don't. Compassion is the most beautiful fashion. When I hear people say it's glamorous or luxurious, I'm at a loss. It would never make me feel that to wear a tortured and killed animal's fur. I am certain it looked better on them. A pair of Chanel sunglasses does the trick for me.

For my toddler, I go for Tom's shoes, and then a needy kid, too, gets a pair or Converse slip-ons. She also has a cute collection of nonleather dress shoes, flip-flops, and sandals. We are also big Converse fans for tennis shoes.

As she gets older, I will explain to her why some items are not worthy of our money. I will tell her that some are made from animals. We don't support that, so we can keep looking to find a better product made by a company who loves animals as we do.

The more people that demand fashion without killing animals, the more high-end and mainstream designers will make alternatives to leather—simple supply and demand. Can you imagine people comparing beautiful products by how ethically they were made instead of by price tag and brand name? I can because when I find a new company making cool vegan fashion, I get a charge from finding the item and then a second charge that I am supporting an ethical company. I get a positive jolt. Most likely, I have saved money and I am supporting a company that is in line with my worldview and values.

You will never see this vegan in hemp or Birkenstocks. Not that there is anything wrong with that, but I love glamour and style. I am Mildred's granddaughter and she passed the torch to me. She also passed along many fur coats even though she knew I would never wear them. I intend to donate them in a thoughtful way. I'll keep the gorgeous 1940s raincoat and many other items to pass along to my daughter. Animal skin and fur as fashion has to come to an end in my family.

Fashion is fun and creative, but it can say even more about you. Let it say that you care while looking fabulous.

The Perfect Vegan

> It's not about being a saint.
> It's about deal breakers.

Living a vegan lifestyle isn't about perfection or feeling high and mighty. It's about choices and being informed. I was no different than a lot of people when it came to loving cheese and a good pair of designer shoes until I discovered the deal breakers.

Most vegans used to eat chicken, for instance. I certainly did—and way too much of it. What made me stop eating chicken for good? When I first saw footage of the chickens in big industrial buildings. Just that alone felt wrong and unnatural to me. That was a deal breaker. What happened to life on a grassy farm in Iowa like in my childhood? This looked like a prison; they were on top of one another, with no room to move. When I did further research, I found out their beaks were sliced off with no painkillers so they couldn't peck at each other from pure frustration and anxiety. That is a serious deal breaker. I remembered back to the film *Baraka* shown in my college philosophy class and that one image of the baby chicks going into the grinder by the thousands. The males are worthless because they cannot produce eggs, so they go into a grinder alive. These facts made eating chicken altogether unappetizing to me. Nothing about this process was humane or just to the animals. It was all about greed and money for the companies, and the consumer was footing the bill. I couldn't pay for animals to be tortured. I had to stop.

Many vegans have eaten steak. I have and even ordered it medium rare. Now, when I see a steak, I see downed cows being pulled by trucks and hoisted by cranes. I have seen this so many times that it is imprinted on my brain. They can be sick and in horrible pain, and still they are prodded and pushed around to go down the line to be killed for food. This is wrong on several levels. For one, this is not humane treatment and number two, many of these animals that end up on your plate are sick.

Additionally, prior to all this, they were shot up with hormones and antibiotics. The business of "beef" is a cruel and filthy business. Cows are very peaceful creatures, and it doesn't make sense to me. This was easy to give up. The entire idea of it was a deal breaker for me once I knew all the facts.

Dairy is a tricky one because people will say, "Well, it's not killing the animal because it's just their milk." I wish that were the case, but it's not. Here's how it goes: The mother cow is artificially inseminated, and when she has her baby, if it's a male calf, it will go into a veal crate and be killed very young. The mother has to endure her baby being taken away from her and is not allowed to feed her own calf. She is hooked to machines that are very painful to give the milk meant for her baby to humans. I have a special disdain for the dairy business. Taking a baby from a mother and stealing the baby's milk is the lowest of the low in my book. When I gave birth to my daughter, I can tell you that my yearning to feed my baby was primal and relentless. My baby wasn't the best sucker in the beginning and I agonized over it. It's not rational but instinctual and very intense. I believe that every mother has the right to feed and be with her young. The dairy business defies that; therefore, I could never support them in any way. Splitting up mothers and babies and stealing a baby's milk should be the definition of a deal breaker.

My life as a vegan is not about perfection. It's more about deal breakers and the fact that I don't feel right paying for someone else to be harmed. I don't have some amazing willpower or the desire to be a saint, but I do have a conscience, and with that comes a line I don't wish to cross. Hurting and murdering animals for a sandwich or a pair of shoes is not who I am, and I will not let someone else make me that. Not a company, not a cultural standard, not my upbringing or conditioning—nothing. I can get what I want and desire without killing or paying someone else to do it.

Find out the process of how products are made, or, in the case of meat and dairy, how they are treated and then killed, and see if there are any deal breakers for you.

Corporations Can Evolve

It's time for them to take notice of vegans

I visit Starbucks almost every morning for my soy latte. I do appreciate that they carry soymilk, and it's the main reason I go. However, they are missing five to seven opportunities each week to sell me other items. In the morning, I would love a vegan croissant or muffin. It is not difficult to make these items without butter or eggs. I often do it at home for my family. I love Starbucks, and especially the quick drive-through, because I have a very busy lifestyle. Not to mention that many times I have three dogs and a toddler in my car, so going in is not an option. If they had anything vegan for my daughter, I would buy it. Dog treats—also vegan—I would want those as well.

Starbucks and many other corporations are missing out. I am an easy mark when it comes to making my girl, my husband, and my pooches happy, but I will not compromise on cruelty.

For lunch, I would spend my money on some sliced veggies with hummus, or tofu and a veggie bowl. The problem is that such products don't exist at Starbucks. It is hard for me to understand why they don't offer vegan items for me and the other millions of us worldwide.

I would also love to see almond milk offered, and an unsweetened version would go over well, because many people are watching the sugar these days.

It's not just me. As I mentioned, I also have a vegan husband who loves pastry, and a toddler who sees the cake pops and wants one, but I tell her no because they are made with dairy and we don't support cruelty to animals. It seems that Starbucks could offer one cruelty-free option at the very minimum, especially for children.

McDonald's lost my business years ago because they don't offer anything vegan but instead feature a menu mostly based on animals being harmed, and that is very unappetizing to me. Burger King gained points in my book for having the veggie burger and sticking with it. It must do well because it is offered all over the United States. I would love to see some nonanimal chicken nuggets added to the list. That would be a smart next step for BK. I would buy those and some sweet potato fries.

I keep waiting for a nationwide pizza company to get wise and offer a vegan pizza. The number of pizzas I have *not* ordered but instead made at home amount to quite a bit of cash especially if you add up all the vegan pizza lovers and the lactose-intolerant people. In one year's time, these pizza chains have said no to lots of money.

Ordering pizza to be delivered is something I would love to do, but someone has to offer a pizza for vegans. I am waiting, and so are lots of other folks. I wonder who will be smart enough to do it first?

Whole Foods does offer vegan pizza by the slice, and I love it. I sure wish more pizza joints had this option so I could pop in and grab a slice when on the road, doing my busy day activities. I love pizza with Daiya or Follow Your Heart vegan cheese.

Another American tradition that needs to get a makeover for the twenty-first century is popcorn. I want it, but not with butter. I want it air-popped with olive oil and salt. This isn't difficult. Vegans and nonvegans will order this healthier version. Popcorn at the movie theaters needs a serious update.

So many corporations are missing the boat in a big way. Vegans want products, minus the cruelty, with emphasis on flavor and health. These companies could hurt animals less, help people to be healthier, and make more money. It's a no-brainer, and everyone wins.

Here are a few more honorable mentions. Dodger's Stadium has a veggie Dodger dog, and for several years now. Not to mention that last time I was in their restaurant, many plant-based dishes were offered. Another reason to say, "Go, Dodgers!"

I am not sure what the Alternative Baking Company is doing right besides making beyond-delicious vegan cookies, but they are in airports across the United States and even in movie theaters. Maybe I should call them to make a vegan popcorn.

I am seeing lots of change, but I say "Let's speed it up a bit." Some of these corporations are really disappointing. The support from nonvegans or transitioning vegans would be wonderful as well. I cannot see any reason why every person wouldn't support more cruelty-free options in the world. If you are opposed to it, please ask yourself why and take a look at your answers. If something still tastes good and is a healthier option, why wouldn't you try it? Not to mention you'd be helping to diminish animal cruelty in the process. Animals deserve more consideration. They are living, breathing, and feeling beings, not products.

When you want to see change, you have to take matters into your own hands and do something. It's important to stand up for what you believe in and ask for what you want. I hope Starbucks and many other companies will evolve and include vegans; but if they don't, we can take our business elsewhere.

One company that is so smart and going to pick up the slack for the other lacking ones is Veggie Grill.

Animal cruelty for profit is on the way out, but how quickly is dependent on all of us.

Vegans and Activism

What are they fighting for?

I know it must seem to some that vegans are fighting everyone. Most vegans oppose the circus, zoos, aquariums and ocean-life parks like SeaWorld. Did you see the film *Blackfish*? If you missed it, I highly recommend it. How could anyone think it is okay to take a baby whale from his mother in the wild and then hold him prisoner for thirty years to make money? Once you see the entire story, the picture looks different. Vegans oppose factory farming and animals used as fabric in fashion. This may seem like a lot to some people, but it boils down to one thing. Vegans are against the cruelty and murder of innocent animals. Sure, there are other good reasons to live a vegan life such as better health, better use of resources, and less harmful impact on our planet. Still, at the heart of veganism is a love and respect for the other beings we share life with on this earth.

Here's the thing, once your compassionate side is really awakened you will see and even feel the suffering of animals and people in all kinds of situations that maybe you hadn't noticed in the past. I know that may seem scary, but it's also amazing because you will see more beauty and truth in the world as well. I cannot guarantee any of this, but it is what happened for me.

As a child, I visited all the places that I protest against now, just like most people. I thought they were the places that animal lovers gathered.

Zoos seemed so cool because you get to see animals that you wouldn't get to see up close otherwise. It never occurred to me that this experience for us came with a huge price for the animals. Most are taken from their families as babies; some are born into captivity and then they are shuffled all around to different places and separated at the will of the humans in charge. Most of the animals are meant to have miles and miles to roam but end up in a small space for their entire life. It's jail for animals. The only difference between zoos and human jails is that they committed no crime. Their misery is making money for a few humans and amusing many others, but is it right? Should an animal's entire life be sacrificed to amuse us? I know the word *research* is thrown around a lot, but the best research and most accurate data regarding animals could be compiled by observing them in their natural habitat.

I have a daughter and I would love for her to see elephants and lions, but I don't feel we need to see them doing unnatural tricks that took years of chaining them down and depriving them of food to achieve. Do I feel my daughter is missing out? Absolutely not! Holding them captive is unnatural, and animals are beautiful, interesting, and hilarious without any of these tricks and silly shows.

Many vegans attend protests, not all. Some vegans don't get into activism, but I do and I will tell you why.

When I think of innocent animals being held captive to be killed in horrific ways, my blood boils and my heart races wanting to help them. When I think of animals being held in scientific labs for years and years, enduring excruciatingly painful tests, I want to free them from this agony. These animals have no voice and are being used and abused; I cannot ignore it and stay silent. I feel sorry for the animal lovers that don't find a way to help animals or stop eating them, wearing them, and paying for the services that torture them. I was once that kind of animal lover and I was not living an authentic life. Once I connected all the dots, it changed me as a person for the better and I got happier. I used to have a lot of self-loathing probably because I was a giant hypocrite.

Vegans such as myself may be hard to take sometimes. I understand that, but the intention is to help, protect, and care for others. You cannot do that by being meek and sitting in the background.

When you see protests regarding animals, I hope you will take a moment to ask, "What are they fighting for?" You might find it a very worthy cause if you took the time.

Five Days of Vegan Meals

A Starter Guide for the Aspiring or Beginner Vegan

This five-day plan is for the new or aspiring vegan. These meals are great transitional meals. They are also great to serve to your meat- and cheese-loving friends.

This is a good start and won't send your friends and family running for the hills because many of these meals are reminiscent of what many American people already eat.

You can indulge and have comfort food without harming animals and with a more nutrient-rich and healthy twist.

Breakfast

1. Tofu scramble – Mash 1/2 container of firm tofu (press water out between 2 napkins over the sink) lightly with a fork in a bowl so it looks a bit like scrambled eggs. Add 1 tsp. dried mustard, 2 tablespoons of nutritional yeast flakes, 1 tablespoon of low sodium tamari (or low sodium soy sauce). Mix in bowl. Spray frying pan with olive oil. Cook on medium heat. Add tomatoes

or spinach, mushrooms, green peppers. or whatever veggies you like in an omelet.

2. Oatmeal – Add blueberries, raspberries or bananas, or all. A little raw sugar or vanilla soymilk never hurts.
3. Breakfast Sandwich – Veggie sausage patties (microwave 2 for one minute) on whole grain bread (toasted) with Daiya cheddar melted on the bread in the toaster oven.
4. Pancakes or waffles (Whole Foods has vegan ones) – 100% maple syrup and fruit of your choice.
5. Protein smoothie – Almond milk, (Plant Fusion and Whole Foods have an amazing vanilla bean and chocolate vegan protein powder), one banana, ice, peanut butter, and chopped dates.

Lunch

1. Tacos – Fry meatless ground round, tomatoes, diced green or red peppers, onions, black beans, and taco spices in a pan. Have shredded lettuce and sliced avocado in two separate bowls. Warm up corn tortillas in a pan. Add first ingredients to the tortilla and top with avocado, shredded lettuce, and salsa.

2. Veggie burger and sweet potato fries – Just do a veggie burger as you would a regular one but make sure to put all of your favorite condiments and lettuce and tomato, or whatever you normally love, to make it great. Bake 8–10 sweet potato fries. Keep portions reasonable if you are watching or wanting to lose weight.

3. Big chopped salad – Go all out. Get good lettuce and chop up all your favorite things. Add garbanzo beans, avocado, green pepper, olives, sliced-up Morningstar chicken nuggets, and some shredded Daiya cheese. I love a dressing called Goddess by Annie's brand. It's delish and vegan. Be creative. Salad can be amazing if it contains what you love. Find a dressing that is not ridiculously high in sodium or sugar that you love. You will start to really dig salads.

4. Eggless salad sandwiches – Mash 1/2 container of firm tofu (press water out) in a bowl, like the omelet. Add 2 tsp. pickle relish, 2 tbsp. of vegan mayo, 1 tsp. mustard, 1/4 tsp. cumin, 1/4 tsp. turmeric, 1/4 tsp. garlic powder, a little diced onion, if you like onions. Mix in bowl; no cooking needed. Toast whole grain bread, slice tomato and lettuce, and make your sandwich.

5. Tortilla pizza – You can use your oven or a toaster oven. Use 2 or 3 small tortillas. First, put marinara sauce, veggies and veggie pepperoni or sausage. Then add Daiya mozzarella on top, put on a cookie sheet, and bake in the oven or on tin foil in the toaster oven.

Dinner

Dinner is so important when trying to eat healthy and maintain a healthy weight. Do you own a steamer that you put in a big saucepan or spaghetti pot? If not, get one. They are only seven dollars at grocery stores or kitchen supply companies. Steaming veggies several times per week is a good way to up the veggies in your life. A little olive oil and nutritional yeast flakes and a sprinkle of sea salt, and you are there. It's simple and tasty.

Try to keep dinner down to veggies and some protein whenever possible.

1. Steamed veggies and quinoa – Cook quinoa like rice, then add nutritional yeast flakes and olive oil or Earth Balance and a touch of salt. With steaming, you just put water in the bottom of the pot, insert the steamer, and put in any veggies you like and steam until somewhat soft. You can also use Earth Balance and nutritional yeast flakes to give a cheesy flavor.

2. Stuffed Green peppers – Get two large green peppers. Cut the tops off but keep

the top as little hats for the pepper. Hallow out the pepper. In a big bowl, mix vegan ground round, tomato sauce, diced mushrooms, onions, carrots, tomatoes and spinach, pinch of garlic salt, pinch of cayenne pepper, and 2 tsp. olive oil. Mix all together and stuff the peppers. Put the tops back on and bake at 425 degrees for about 35–45 minutes, depending on the oven.

3. Veggie Chili – You will need 2 cans kidney beans, 1 large can of tomato juice, 2 tsp. olive oil, 6–8 garlic cloves, 1 medium carrot (diced),1 medium stalk of celery (diced), 2 tsp. cumin, 2 tsp. basil, 2 tsp. chili powder, 1 tsp. salt, 1 medium green pepper (diced), 1 medium can of tomatoes, and 3 tsp. of tomato paste. Sauté all veggies in a frying pan and start pouring the tomato juice and spices in a big pot. Then add all veggies to the pot and simmer for about 30–40 minutes. When served, add Daiya cheese and parsley on top. With canned items, always go for the lowest sodium and sugar content. Read the labels.

4. Faux chicken nuggets and steamed green beans – To make green beans more amazing, sauté with a little tamari or low sodium soy sauce and garlic.

5. Spaghetti with marinara sauce and green olives and a nice salad – Try the spaghetti

that is made from quinoa. Dice the green olives. Add 2 garlic cloves and sauté with the marinara. It's a simple dish but really good. Only make 1/2 the spaghetti and don't eat all of that. Save a little for lunch the next day. Eat your salad first so you aren't as hungry. Whenever you eat pasta, just keep the portion smaller and always eat a salad first.

Snacks

- Nuts
- Edamame (soybeans in the pod) – warm and put a little salt and tamari to taste
- Fruit
- Peanut butter with celery
- Hummus and carrots
- Seaweed crisps
- Kale chips

Once you get into some of these food items, your body will start to crave them. You will be surprised.

Busy Mama: On-the-Go Recipes

Bruschetta

Shopping List

Spices

    1/2 tsp. salt

    1/2 tsp. freshly ground pepper

Produce

    5 medium Roma tomatoes

    3 cloves garlic

    1/2 lemon juice

    1 cup fresh basil

Additional Ingredients

    1 baguette

    1/4 cup olive oil

To Prepare

Combine all ingredients except lemon juice. Pour over tomatoes. Add lemon last and serve over very lightly toasted and sliced baguette.

Collard Green Wraps

Shopping List

Produce

4–6 whole collard green leaves

fresh mushrooms, sliced

1 red pepper

1 onion

2–4 garlic cloves, minced

Additional Ingredients

ponzu sauce

sunflower oil

Smart Ground, 1 package

hot chili sauce (optional)

To Prepare

Sauté mushrooms, red peppers, onions, and garlic in sunflower oil and Ponzu sauce. Add veggie Smart Ground round after veggies are sautéed. Mix all up and simmer. Place ingredients on collard green leaves and top with hot chili sauce. Wrap the collard greens like a taco and enjoy.

Dea's Cioppino

Shopping List

Spices

    2 tbsp. dried oregano

    1 tsp. red chili flakes

    2 tbsp. tarragon

Fresh Herbs

    2 tbsp. parsley (fresh)

    1/4 cup basil (fresh)

Produce

    5 garlic cloves, minced

    2 red bell peppers, diced

    2 onions, diced

    5 large tomatoes, diced

    1 1/2–2 lbs. oyster mushrooms (fresh)

Liquids

    2 tbsp. olive oil

    1 1/2 cups white wine

    6 cups low sodium vegetable broth

Miscellaneous

1 vegetable bouillon cube

To Prepare

In a skillet, sauté garlic, red peppers, onions, tomatoes, and oyster mushrooms in olive oil for approximately 5 minutes.

In a large pot, combine all liquids, spices, and miscellaneous.

Add ingredients from skillet and simmer for 30 minutes on ultra-low heat.

Gazpacho

Shopping List

Spices

- 1 tsp. basil
- 1 tsp. tarragon
- 1/2 tsp. cumin
- 1 tsp. sea salt
- 1 tsp. fresh ground black pepper
- 1/2 tsp. cayenne (optional)

Produce

- 1/4 cup parsley
- 3–4 garlic cloves, minced
- 1/2 cup onion, minced
- 2 scallions, minced
- 1 red pepper, minced
- 1 medium cucumber, minced
- 2 cups tomatoes, diced

Additional Ingredients

- 5 cups tomato juice
- 2 tbsp. olive oil
- 1/4 cup white wine or wine vinegar

To Prepare

Combine all.

Serve as is for a chunky Gazpacho or purée for a smooth gazpacho.

Party Noodles

Shopping List

Produce

- 1 package of cabbage slaw
- 1 bunch green onions

Additional Ingredients

- 2 packages dried Asian noodles
- 1 cup sesame seeds
- 1/2 cup slivered almonds
- 1/2 cup olive oil
- 1/3 cup cider vinegar
- 1/2 tsp. of a vegetable bouillon cube
- 1/2 cup sugar

To Prepare

Crush up the dried noodles, add sesame seeds and almonds, and set aside.

Chop the green onions very small and add to the cabbage slaw.

To make dressing

Mix 1/2 cup, 1/2 cup oil, 1/3 cup cider vinegar, 1/2 tsp vegetable bouillon. Keep dressing in separate bowl.

Combine the dry ingredients and the dressing in a large bowl just before serving to your guests.

Perfect Puttanesca

Shopping List

Spices

- red pepper flakes
- salt and pepper

Produce

- 8 oz. of zucchini, cut in 1/4 inch half moons
- 4 garlic cloves, finely chopped
- 12 basil leaves, rolled and sliced thinly
- 4 fresh Roma tomatoes, diced
- lemon, juiced

Additional Ingredients

- 2/3 cup kalamata olives
- 2 tbsp. capers
- 1 small can pear tomatoes
- 1 pound penne, cooked al dente
- vegan parmesan
- olive oil

To Prepare

Sauté zucchini, garlic, tomato, and capers in olive oil for about 7 minutes. Then add all other ingredients, pasta last, and top with salt, pepper, red pepper flakes, and vegan parmesan.

Raw Tunot Salad

Shopping List

Produce

- carrots
- celery
- lettuce
- sun-dried tomatoes

Additional Ingredients

- cashews
- tabouli
- nondairy mayo (Follow Your Heart)
- 2 tsp. dressing (green garlic)

To Prepare

Put carrots, celery, cashews, and Tabouli in the small food processor really fast (you don't want it too chopped up). Then add one tbsp. of nondairy mayo and 2 tsp. green raw dressing. I like green garlic. This is the middle scoop (like a tuna fish). Then do a chopped salad to your liking for the rest.

Stuffed Peppers

Shopping List

Spices

- 1 tsp. Italian seasoning
- 1/4 tsp. cayenne pepper
- 1/4 tsp. salt
- 1 pinch black pepper

Produce

- 4 peppers
- 1 medium onion, chopped
- 2 garlic cloves, minced
- 1 small tomatoes, chopped

Additional Ingredients

- 2 packages of Smart Ground
- 1 8 oz. can tomato sauce
- 1/4 cup bread crumbs (optional)
- 1/2 cup vegan mozzarella (Daiya)
- 1 tbsp. vegan Parmesan cheese

To Prepare

Cut tops off the peppers and clean out. Save tops to place back on like little hats. In a large bowl, combine all ingredients except the mozzarella and Parmesan cheese. Mix ingredients well and stuff the peppers. Bake at 350 degrees for 30–35 minutes. Take the peppers out of the oven and top first with the mozzarella and then sprinkle with the Parmesan. Bake for another 5–7 minutes. Put the tops back on and serve. It's a great presentation. You can also slice the peppers into long strips and let the inside just fall on top and serve that way.

Tofu Breakfast Scramble

Shopping List

Spices

>1 tsp. dried mustard
>
>sea salt
>
>pepper

Produce

>2 small Roma tomatoes
>
>fresh spinach
>
>cremini mushrooms, diced
>
>1 green pepper
>
>any veggies you love

Additional Ingredients

>1 container firm tofu
>
>2 tbsp. nutritional yeast flakes
>
>1 tbsp. low sodium tamari
>
>1 tsp. sunflower, olive, or canola oil

To Prepare

The most important thing with the tofu scramble is to get the water out of the tofu. I have a tofu press (Tofuxpress.

com, $50). I highly recommend it. However, you can achieve almost the same result pressing the tofu between two napkins.

The next step is to mash it with a fork until it has the consistency similar to scrambled eggs.

Spray skillet with canola oil. On low heat, add spices, tamari, oil, and yeast flakes. Add the veggies and let simmer on low heat for a few minutes before adding the mashed tofu.

Lastly, cook as lightly or well-done, or as you desire.

Trees and Nuts Salad

Shopping List

produce

broccoli

red onion

Additional ingredients

walnuts

sunflower seeds

vinegar

veganaise

sugar

To prepare

Steam broccoli. Add sunflower seeds, walnuts, and sliced red onion in a large bowl.

In a small bowl, mix 1/2 cup veganaise, 3 tbsp. sugar, and a bit of vinegar.

Mix all together and add more of whatever you like.

Vegan Spaghetti Bolognese

Shopping List

Spices

    1 tsp. oregano, dried

    1 tsp cayenne pepper

    1 tsp. basil, dried

    sea salt and freshly ground pepper to taste

Produce

    1 green pepper, finely diced

    1 onion, finely diced

    4 garlic cloves, minced

Additional Ingredients

Yves Smart Ground or any soy-based ground protein vegetable bouillon cube

1 tsp. vegan Worcestershire sauce

can of chopped tomatoes in purée

small can sliced black olives

1/2 tsp. sugar

dried spaghetti (either Italian spaghetti or quinoa Spaghetti)

To Prepare

In skillet, sauté green pepper, onion, and garlic cloves in olive oil. Add all spices. When green pepper looks tender, add Smart Ground, vegetable bouillon cube, Worcestershire sauce, can of tomatoes, canned olives, and sugar.

In large pot, boil spaghetti with a pinch of salt and dash of olive oil. Spaghetti is best al dente, so don't over cook. Should be soft but with a slight bite in the center.

When spaghetti is finished, add Bolognese sauce on top.

Ladies Lunching Sandwiches

1. Mash 2 avocados and add 1 cup fresh or frozen steamed peas. Add 1 tsp. lemon juice and spread on nice fancy bread or regular with the crust cut. Add sliced tomatoes or radishes.

2. Prepare a sliced avocado and a sliced tomato. Spread tomato, basil, and hummus on both sides.

3. Arrange in layers: almond butter and thinly sliced banana, and then drizzle dark chocolate.

4. Arrange in layers: Tofurky peppered deli slices, thinly sliced green peppers, and sundried tomato paste

A Few Fun Tricks

Every parent knows that at times children assert their independence by refusing to eat what you prepare for them. I make sure to offer my daughter balanced meals, but I also cleverly include extra nutrients into the things I know she will eat. Here are a few of my latest tricks.

Brownies

> vegan brownie mix
>
> 1 can black beans
>
> 1/2 cup almond milk

Strain black beans and refill the can with fresh water. Blend in blender, water and all. Put all in a large bowl and stir until smooth.

Bake according to instructions on the box.

Peanut Butter Cookies

> 1 cup peanut butter
>
> 1/2 cup applesauce
>
> 1 1/4 cup sugar
>
> 1/4 cup vanilla soymilk
>
> 1 egg replacer
>
> 1 cup flour
>
> 3/4 cup baking soda

1/2 cup garbanzo beans

375 degrees for 12 minutes

Crisscross with fork

Amazing Popcorn

Pop your corn with no butter.

When done, spray lightly with canola oil, nutritional yeast flakes, and a little salt. Best popcorn ever. Add sriracha for adults who like a little kick.

Nutritional Yeast Flakes

I use them to make mac and cheese. Just add a little oil, water, and the flakes.

They are great for casseroles, pasta dishes, and veggies.

My tofu scramble (featured in the recipe section) would not be the same without it.

Flaxseed Oil

This is high in Omega 3. I put a teaspoon in my daughter's juice a couple times a week.

Hemp Seeds

These are high in protein. I keep them in a shaker by the stove.

The Holidays

From Halloween to Christmas

The holidays are a good time to vote for what you believe in with your money. Every dollar you spend is a message, and we all spend *a lot* during these three months.

I am obviously against any animal cruelty, and I show that with the money I spend on food, clothing, gifts, cleaning products, skincare, etc., I hope more and more people will stop to think what they are voting for when they spend their money.

Your money is your voice to companies, not only regarding your preferences but what you will tolerate and support in terms of how they do business. Collectively, it's our power, so use it wisely. Support companies that are in line with your values.

Halloween

I love this holiday. It's fun to dress up or at least dress up my kid and go around and look at all the freaks.

Believe it or not, there are many unintentional vegan candies to choose from and intentional vegan "everything" is on the rise, so there are many choices.

Here's a short list.

Vegan Candy

- Blow Pops
- Cry Babies
- Dark Chocolate (many vegan brands)
- Dots
- Dum-Dums
- Lemonheads
- Sour Patch Kids
- Swedish Fish
- Sweet Tarts
- Twizzlers

My daughter knows which products are vegan and which ones hurt animals. For instance, she knows she can have Oreo cookies sometimes and Lay's potato chips because they are unintentionally vegan. She already knows the good and the bad products by the packages.

We are lucky because we have many vegan friends who will have vegan candy for trick or treat night.

I give out vegan candy to the little goblins and superheroes that come to my door, and they don't even notice the difference.

As far as holidays go, Halloween is the easy one.

Thanksgiving

My family does a Tofurky roast every year. We love it. Some people don't care for it. There are so many different vegan roasts now that each person should try them all.

We just happen to love Tofurky, and we have tried many over the years. My husband gets very into it and marinates overnight. He has a whole mixture of olive oil, soy sauce, garlic, and onions. He makes mushroom gravy and the stuffing for the roast. I make green bean casserole and mashed potatoes and a few different vegetable dishes. I usually buy a vegan pumpkin pie from Whole Foods to be honest. I did make one a few years ago, and it wasn't great. I like to cook, but baking is tedious to me. We have a big feast just as everyone does, minus the dead bird in the middle of the table.

We do go to my cousins in Arizona or my in-laws in Ohio once every few years, so we simply bring our Tofurky roast or have it delivered. It's not a big deal. I prefer to be home during the holidays at my own house with my dogs, but it is nice to see family too.

Christmas

I do enjoy Christmas even though the whole shopping thing gets overwhelming. I don't love shopping, especially in crowds, so I try to do it early.

We do a fake tree and love it. We used to do a small potted tree and then plant it in the yard after, and let me tell you, our yard in Venice oddly had many evergreen trees. We graduated to the big fake tree. I think it's better for us. I do bake cookies and decorate them for my daughter, but I don't go overboard. We love our Tofurky roast, so sometimes we do another one on Christmas. We change it up. We are festive. The only thing that is really different food-wise, just like Thanksgiving, is the dead animal in the middle of the table. We don't use dairy butter, but oils instead, like coconut, canola, or olive oil. Soy or almond milk instead of dairy milk; and no eggs, so egg replacer or banana or flaxseeds in place of eggs.

I hope this makes you realize that it's not that big of a deal or unmanageable to be vegan during the holidays. The most annoying part for new vegans are the comments from rigid family members or rude friends who strive to make you feel bad or awkward. For some reason, you wanting to be compassionate toward animals and be healthier offends them. This is more about them than you. Just ride it out and keep your sense of humor or tell them off, if that is your style. Just kidding! Kind of. I've done both, so maybe mix it up for variety. Seriously though, keep your cool, have a glass of wine, and enjoy yourself.

Happy holidays!

Films

I highly recommend these films:

1. Forks Over Knives
2. The Ghosts in our Machine
3. Earthlings
4. An Inconvenient Truth
5. Food Inc.
6. Vegucated
7. Fat, Sick and Nearly Dead
8. Bold Native
9. Blackfish
10. The Cove
11. Dealing Dogs.
12. Skin Trade

Please check out my own short film, *Harmony Drive*, on Youtube.

Books

Some amazing books to check out:

1. *The Mad Cowboy*
   by Howard Lyman
2. *The China Study*
   by T. Colin Campbell
3. *The New Good Life*
   by John Robbins
4. *Diet for a New America*
   by John Robbins
5. *How to Go Further*
   by Woody Harrelson and Friends
6. *Slaughterhouse*
   by Gail Eisnitz

Recipe books:

1. *Skinny Bitch in the Kitch*
   by Rory Freedman and Kim Barnouin
2. *Moosewood Cookbook*
   by Mollie Katzen
3. *Blissful Bites*
   by Christy Morgan

4. *The New Vegan Cookbook*
   by Lorna Sass
5. *Vegan Deli*
   by Joanne Stepaniak

Children's books:
1. *Vegan Is Love*
   by Ruby Roth
2. *V Is for Vegan*
   by Ruby Roth
3. *That's Why We Don't Eat Animals*
   by Ruby Roth

Printed in the USA
CPSIA information can be obtained
at www.ICGtesting.com
LVHW022131041023
760082LV00002B/12